"Why Me?"

"Why Me?"

A True Story of Wanda (Rankin) Lawhorn's
Will To Survive Four Types of Cancer

Dr. Tmar

To order additional copies of this book, contact:
Xlibris Corporation
1-888-795-4274
www.Xlibris.com
Orders@Xlibris.com
79382

Contents

Dedication

I dedicate this book to all Cancer survivors, non-Cancer survivors, their families and friends and all that have been involved with this dreaded disease.

Wanda (Rankin) Lawhorn.

"The Daffodil"

When Spring arrives, and you know it will,
You will be looking at the Daffodil.

They come in yellow, and they come in white,
People do not realize, they're here for a fight.

They look like a horn, and sound like one too,
They are sent by God to watch over you.

The Daffodil, is the Spring Cancer Flower,
They bring hope, each second, minute and hour.

When you see the Daffodil, looking so strong,
Please remember to pray along.

A prayer for Spring that it comes each year,
The Daffodil will stand tall and never have fear.

Spring is the beginning, and not the end,
Never say goodbye to your dearest friend.

Dr. Tmar,
Teresa May Raley

Introduction

If you think it is hard to climb Mt. Everest, or dive to the deepest depths of the ocean or ride the wildest bull in captivity or even be in a hurricane or tornado, survive a flood or fire, you don't know anything until you have survived four different types of Cancer.

The very sound of this word especially if you have had it sends chills down your spine, not to mention what it does to your stomach and your mind.

No one knows what this word can do to you when you are told that you have cancer. Your thoughts are, my whole life is instantly over. You just know from that point on death is inevitable. The doctors usually are cold about it when they deliver the message, after you are stunned they proceed with your options and before you leave their office that day you are so confused, you don't remember anything they have told you except we found a mass and you have Cancer.

From then on you have numerous testing, run here and there trying to get everything done before your treatments start. Your whole world now is like a merry go round.

Live my experience, live my inner most feelings and share my every thought, then ask yourself: Why Me?

Travel with me on my journey of 49 years living with these Cancers.

Cervical, Hodgins Lymphoma, Squamous Cell Carcinoma and Single Cell Carcinoma.

Teresa May Raley,
Dr. Tmar

Chapter One

The Beginning

When your eyes opens for the first time and your lungs are breathing fresh air, and everyone in the delivery room is rushing to keep you alive you never realize at this time how your life will change once you leave this room. This was me December 29, 1950 4:05 p.m. I was born in the worst snow storm of the year, at Miner's Hospital in Frostburg, Maryland, it was a total blizzard. If I had waited a few days more I may have missed the storm. Being born under Capricorn ruler of Time, I could not wait. Little did I know how my life would change as I aged. I know I had most child hood diseases but at that point I was pretty young and strong.

I was as proud as a peacock, I was the first child, the first daughter and the first granddaughter, I thought everyone was happy for me, but I soon found out my father Frederick was not proud at all. He didn't hide his feelings that his preference would have been a bouncing baby boy. I could feel that his love for me did not exist. He never held me or gave me comfort, I really felt sad for him. This so called love soon turned to abuse and torment. My mom pretty well went along with it, I think maybe she was afraid of him, I knew he drank a lot. If it hadn't been for my wonderful grandmother Mary I don't know what I would have done. She was always taking up for me, her and Pap. I just never understood my father's hatred.

My brother William (Bill) was born June 30, 1953, my father was ecstatic with joy, he finally had the son he always wanted. I accepted by brother. I was so glad to have a friend and a playmate, at least it took some of the attention from me. I noticed Bill was always brought gifts home from work from our dad, I felt sad but I didn't expect it for me because I never got gifts anyway. My father treated Bill so much better.

When I was nine years old, we were living in a small town in western Maryland, when a knock came to the door, it was the police, my father had been in a bad car accident and he had been killed instantly. Him and a friend had been drinking and celebrating the friend's birthday. The friend had just gotten new tires for the car and he wanted to try them out. Together they left the bar and proceeded to travel at a very high rate of speed. When they approached a very sharp turn they were going so fast that the car left the road, hit a culvert, and became airborne, they were killed immediately, their possessions and car parts were found everywhere.

My most vivid memory at that point was the doll baby that my father had given me for a gift when I was a small child. That was the only gift I ever remember him giving me. That and the abuse.

At age eleven I started my menstrual cycle, this was at an early age I thought. I sure wasn't ready for this gift. Every month without fail I experienced unusual pain, vomiting, and passing out, but yet I had hardly any bleeding. In those days your parents didn't take you to the doctor for just anything, you had to be dying, which I thought I was. My mother insisted it would pass.

The pain was so severe that while in school I would be sent home every month because of it. There were many occasions when my mother didn't care for us, or so I thought. Once in the winter, it was so cold, and I had a feeling that there was no school, but as usual our mother said we had to go. My brother and I had to walk a great distance to get to the bus stop, it was up a hill and it felt like the distance you would climb to get to Mt. Everest. We stood at the bus stop for over an hour freezing because we were afraid to go home, because if the bus came and we missed school we would be in even bigger trouble. The bus never came and I ended up with frozen toes. Winters were horrible when we were kids, but as usual mom made us go no matter what, how could she have sent us out in such weather.

Chapter Two

Willie, Born December 19, 1972

Even into my teen years the same symptoms existed, I still had the pain, the passing out and little or no bleeding. I just figured this was normal, so therefore I just ignored the pain and kept on going, Mom wasn't taking me to the doctors, so I would just have to deal with it.

I spent a lot of time at my Grandmas. She was my Nana, she was my world. Bill and I always had to go to Church with Grandpa and Grandma every Friday night and on Sunday. Mom never went she would stay home and run the little country store that Pap and Nana owned. Bill and I had lots of friends in this little town. We would play baseball, basketball, you know all the childhood games, and it was great fun going there, it was a little taste of freedom from where we lived. There was only three houses where we lived, back in the woods, no kids to play with and definitely nothing to do. So going over to Paps and Nana's was special, even if we only got to go over when we went to church. Twice a week was better than nothing.

I had a special friend that lived in the town and we became very close, we were inseparable.

We played sports together, stayed at my house together, talked a lot on the phone and just basically had good clean fun. Her name was Trecia, she was four years, older than me, very athletic and funny. Trecia was kinda like the clown in the town she was always doing something funny or just plain being silly. We got along great and for the first time in my life I had a real friend. I was surprised that my mom took to her so well, she even let her stay at our house. That was unusual because she never left anyone stay over. We would play records, dance and try to sing. We had a lot of fun.

Trecia and I attended the same school and after she graduated she decided to go away to find better work, there wasn't much to do here. I would be turning 18 in December and I asked mom's permission to go with her. I promised I would finish school where ever we ended up. Mom agreed another shocker.

My menstrual cycle was still the same nothing had changed. I still had all the same symptoms.

We stayed in the D.C. area for around 3 years, we both were homesick so home we came bag and baggage. We got a place here and still remained friends. Things got tight money wise and I decided to move back with my mom. That was a mistake, it was like I was her child again.

In 1972 I became interested in Trecia's cousin Wayne, at the time I didn't know he was married, we started dating and the next thing I knew I was pregnant, being with a guy for the first time I was totally unprepared and then when I confronted him about the baby, his first reply was "it's not mine". That hurt was unbearable, to think you would give yourself to a man and then he just walks away. I did my best because I wasn't going to give my child away, I knew my Nana and Pap would be there for me. I was staying with my mom when I met Charles, he lived in Baltimore and in the summer he would come to our area to visit his grandparents, they lived below my mom. Charles and I became friends and soon we were dating, I knew I didn't love him, but I thought I would give it a chance. He knew I was pregnant and that didn't seem to matter to him, he was willing to take the responsibility of me and my unborn child.

Willie G. was born December 19, 1972. My birthday is December 29 and his so called biological fathers was December 9, How about those numbers 9-19-29. His father was never a part of his life.

Willie was a sick baby, he cried constantly for five years. I had him to every doctor I could take him to and no one seemed to know what caused him to cry or why he was crying. He would be playing then he would turn blue and then he would pass out, this was happening all the time, and no one knew why. Maybe he inherited his illness from me, I was always sick, I still hadn't found out what was wrong with me, at least I didn't have the cramps and pain while I was pregnant. Finally Willie was diagnosed with a very serious heart problem, he had a hole in his heart, that was why he kept passing out, and why he would turn blue, he wasn't getting any oxygen. as soon as he had the hole repaired in his heart he stopped crying and passing out. But only God knows how he ever lived for five years. He grew up to be a body builder, you would never know he was sick a day in his life. He is a joy in my life and I love him very much.

—

Chapter Three

January 22, 1974 Melinda

I had been living in Baltimore for close to two years now, it was what I had hoped to accomplish. Life was not what I thought it would be with Charles, he was not the man he promised to be. He drank too much, didn't come home until he felt like it, did drugs and worst of all abused me. On one occasion after he had been out drinking, he came home and while I was bending over the crib to give Willie a bottle, he came up behind me and struck me in the back of the head with a brass lamp. He would leave for days, and as soon as he came home I got a beating he would always wait until I wasn't looking and he would hit me from behind, he never faced me when he beat me. I never went anywhere I had no freedom. He supported us but never gave me any kind of money. When he would leave for days at a time, he would never leave me any money not even to buy diapers. One night he came home drunk and I was upstairs, he came up the steps grabbed my hair (it was very long) wrapped it around his arm like you would wrap spaghetti around a fork and just twisted it as tight as he could, threw me on the bed tore my clothes off and raped me, I did not fight back because I knew it would only make things worse. He totally took advantage of me. I was scared to death of him, and he knew it. He would abuse me for no reason, he would just start beating on me, he didn't have to be drunk, it was like an obsession. sometimes I would look at him the wrong way and he would lose it. I lived in fear for three years being married to him.

In May 1973, I was 24 years old I had made an appointment with my doctor for a check up and I was surprised to find out that I was pregnant. I didn't understand because I had my period the whole time, but then I remembered I had my period the whole time with Willie too. I wanted out of this marriage so bad I could taste it, and now I was having another baby with this mad man, what was I going to do, where was I gonna go with two small children. I couldn't turn to his family and mine lived too far away. My grandparents were older and I couldn't ask them to take me in, besides he would have come there and terrorized them. My mother hated him but she didn't want to get involved either, she kept telling me to leave him, but where was I going to go.

On January 22, 1974 my beautiful daughter Melinda was born. I thought this might make a change in him since he was her biological father, it didn't matter at all, she made no difference, I still got the beatings, he still drank and did what he wanted. I decided to try to make it work because now I had two children and I would have to do what I had to do to raise them.

Charles could be nice if he wasn't drinking, but then when something pissed him off he would be crazy as usual. In December, 1976 He gave me a brand new car for my birthday, Willie had been sick with pneumonia, Charles had made plans for dinner for my birthday, I refused to go because I didn't want to leave Willie with the baby sitter. Of course Charles threw a fit, he started throwing beer bottles through the picture window, I gathered up the kids and left in my new birthday car. That was the best birthday I ever had.

Chapter Four

The Long Road

At last I thought I could breathe again. The kids and I stayed in the car for a few days and then I remembered Charles had a large amount of savings bonds. I was determined to get them, after all he never gave me anything but pure hell. I had been informed that the police had picked him up and he was in jail for throwing the beer bottles through the picture window, I waited my chance and made sure he wasn't home I went inside took all of the bonds and was on my merry way, the second happiest day of my life.

The kids and I found an apartment, it wasn't the best but we made it home, at least we were together and away from that monster. The kids seemed happy, even though we had no furniture they enjoyed playing in the big bundles of clothes that I took with me when we left. This was our kitchen, living room and our beds. I am glad they were so young, if they had been older it might have been hard. Willie was 4 and Melinda was 2. They were such loving children, I knew I had made the right decision to leave. I returned the shiny new birthday present, locked the keys in it and started our new journey. I knew life was only going to get better.

I filed for divorce, what a waste of time, every time we would go to court Charles would protest it. Believe it or not finally after seven long years of his outlandish protesting, the Judge finally granted me a divorce, with child support. How much harder can life be. I was about to find out.

Life was harder than I thought it would be, but we were making it and that's what mattered. I had to work a little harder than most people. I was working three jobs, a bank manager, working for a cleaning company and working in a wallpaper store. I was totally exhausted all the time but I kept going until one day at the age of 32, I was working at the bank and I didn't feel well, I was walking across the floor headed for my desk when I got this horrible pain in my chest, I didn't know what was happening but soon found out it was a heart attack. After being taken to the hospital I found out that I had four blocked arteries. The doctor said it was stress related. The procedure I had done, was angioplasty. It was an opening of the arteries with a balloon. This just added more information to my chart of many accomplishments. I forgot to mention the appendicitis, fatty tumors and twelve broken bones.

I am sure by now you are wondering what happened to Charles. Well he didn't go away. Every time I turned around he was there to remind me that he was still alive and still loved me, but yet he was still abusing me, he would grab me and throw me around, when I would leave work he was always there, it was like he fell out of the sky. He would just show up.

Willie was 10 now and Melinda was 8, they pretty well knew what he was capable of. I knew I just had to ignore him no matter what I couldn't let him get to me.

I lived in the same court with Edwards parents, they were good people and we were all friends. I spent a lot of time talking to Edward, it seemed we had a lot in common. We found ourselves always talking about something. The talking soon turned to dating, then we moved in together. We lived as a married couple for twelve years and then we decided to get married. It only lasted three years when I found him running around with his hair stylist. It was over then, no forgiving, just get the hell out. I guess we were all talked out at this point. I felt he was a good man but I wasn't about to play second fiddle to anyone.

Even though I finally met another man Edward, and had gotten married and divorced Edward, Charles was still hanging around. It took me seven long years to get a divorce from him, every time we went to court he protested the divorce and he never did stopped bugging me. Edward didn't play his games, he spoke to him, treated him decent and just accepted the fact that Charles was there. He knew what kind of a person he was. Edward knew there would be trouble so he just dealt with it. I thought we had a good marriage we seemed to get along, we did things together, hardly ever fought, maybe I was fooling myself. He never worried that I would go back to Charles, he knew how much I despised him.

Edward could have been a good man, I don't know what happened, after three years, he starting having an affair when I found out, the marriage was over. There was no way I was taking him back.

Chapter Five

Here We Go Again

It was time to think about what was happening to me again, I had started losing weight, just started a new job, where there was room for advancement, it was time to cry I was lonely, I lost my second husband and now I just received news that my wonderful, beautiful Nana had passed away. Even though I made it through all the hurt and pain from the past how was I going to live without my Nana in my life. Pap had already passed away earlier. But Nana was my heart and soul, how was I going to accept this.

All the walls were closing in on me, the kids were grown and had moved out on their own, I was all alone except for my cat Fuzzy, she was such a dear pet, I'm so glad I had her to pass the time with. The weight loss kept coming, I figured it was from all the stress that I was enduring. I thought I was eating good working 50 to 60 hours a week and I had unbelievable energy, I couldn't understand how I could keep on going. The weight was still coming off, that was fine, I thought I could lose a little anyway, when I went to bed and checked myself I was the same weight, when I checked myself the next morning, I was shocked I had lost ten pounds over night. How could this be? This was a great way to lose weight or so I thought. The holidays were here now and so I put the weight loss at the back of my mind, I would deal with it later.

In February 1993 I decided to get a check up just to ease my mind. As I was explaining the weight loss the doctor seemed confused. He decided to send me for a mammogram because of my age at that time 42. The test were done and the doctor had some bad news for me. I had an eight inch mass attached to my aorta and esophagus. It was a tumor. Immediately all the testing began, run here do this run there do this, I was so exhausted from the testing, I didn't see how I would ever do the treatment. I had MRIS< CAT SCANS< XRAYS< BLOOD WORK and BIOPSIES., plus I was still trying to work and maintain a life.

All my brain was doing was registering CANCER, that's was all I could think of day and night, even when I tried to sleep my brain would still be processing this horrible thought. My every thought and action revolved around this word. Eighteen years earlier when they found the cervical cancer, I guess I didn't process it the same way. After I had the surgery I didn't have any kind of treatment. No one has any idea what you are going to go through with this terrible disease until you have it. Believe me it's a living Hell.

You sit there and listen, like you know what they are talking about, but all you can hear is Cancer.

I knew in my heart I was gonna die, I had this nonchalant feeling about the whole situation.

They were explaining how they were going to open up my chest for a more evasive biopsy. I told them I didn't want it. I was so sick of test, I wanted to die just from the testing. They insisted on these test so they could see if it was benign, malignant or if it was cancer.

Without any warning the doctor grabbed my cheeks and looked me straight in the eye and told me if you don't have this surgery," you will die" It finally hit me, I guess I better be prepared. I decided to have the surgery and deep in my mind I knew something was going to go wrong. I had nothing on my mind but the Cancer, I knew what it did to people and I wasn't going through it.

When I got home from hearing all the bullshit about the big "C" I looked for my son's 410 shotgun and I was damn well intended on using it. I had it loaded sitting beside me on the couch, I kept staring at it and telling myself I would die either way. Should I do it now or let the Cancer kill me? I heard Willie open the door and come in. "Hey mom," I heard him say. I didn't answer him at first, I didn't want him to see me this way. He came into the living room, saw the gun on the couch and was totally shocked, "Mom" he yelled what are you doing"? I tried to explain how I felt, he didn't want to hear it, he knew I could fight it, he took the gun and left. Every one tells you, you can fight it, but no one knows how big of a battle it really is until you have to go through it. The treatment alone is enough to kill you. Sure it might make you better, but for how long. Have you ever seen a person on tv say, "I'm a Cancer survivor and I have been Cancer free for fifty years." It's your choice, what are you going to do?

My chest was opened from my sternum to my side, under my left breast. The incision was approximately twelve inches long. After closing me with staples, wire, stitches and tape I spent two weeks in the hospital.

After being home for three days, I started to smell this horrible odor, which no`one else even noticed. I was trying to pull myself upright on the sofa when my incision literally exploded, it just popped open, thick green infection flew out of it. I returned to the hospital where the doctor had his office. As soon as he saw me he started to remove all the gadgets that were supposed to be holding me together, (he didn't even give me anything for pain) he had to remove the infection as soon as possible. I was never told but I totally believe the green infection was gangrene. I found out later it was.

After being readmitted to the hospital, every thirty minutes for fourteen days without fail, I was scraped until they finally removed all the infection. The infection was also in my ribs and as a result of this I lost part of one. They closed me up while I waited on the diagnosis, is it Cancer or not. The news finally came, YES, It was Cancer, that was the last thing I wanted to hear. It was diagnosed as Hodgins Lymphoma, what the hell was that? I soon found out it comes from having a weak immune system, it travels through the lymphatic system. I never heard of such a disease, and of course it was inoperative. Now what?

I was informed the mass was so large they were afraid it would shut off my esophagus and cause me to suffocate. They started giving me high doses of chemotherapy. I took eleven pills each day, and on Friday every week after working eight hours a day I would go to the cancer center, and for four hours through a needle in my vein I would be fed a bag of liquid chemotherapy along with a bag of nausea medicine.

I had been out of work for several months, I had no income and no one to help me. The kids had their own lives to worry about and I couldn't ask them for anything. I was devastated I had no money to pay my bills, and the bill collectors didn't want to hear any kind of excuses at all. I had to do something, I wasn't going to live in a car again, even if it was a new one.

I ended up losing my car, and my home. I moved in with my ex husband Edward's mother, she and I always had a good relationship from day one. She never forgave Edward for running around on me. I was so glad I had her. Fuzzy and I were happy there. I just couldn't live off of my ex mother-in law, so I decided to go back to work. The doctor wasn't very happy, he told me with the amount of chemo. I was taking he didn't see how I could work, I insisted that he sign the papers and I returned to work. It was one of the hardest things I have ever done, but I was determined to make it.

My whole body was so out of whack, I had blood clots, they couldn't get my blood regulated, I was put into isolation, I was sick from the chemo. I ate saltine crackers by the box full, they seemed to be the only thing that helped with the nausea. My hair was past my waist when I was diagnosed, soon it began to fall out in hand fulls. When I would take a shower the water would back up in the tub because the hair clogged up the drain. I decided to get it cut, I was lucky for once all my hair didn't fall out. The chemo was to take eight months to complete, then I was to do fourteen days straight of radiation to my chest it would end on my birthday, another wonderful gift.

Chapter Six

Personal Feelings

When my treatment ended in December, I was informed that the tumor had shrunk, it was now the size of a fifty cent piece, I felt real good about that considering when I started treatment it was eight inches in diameter. I was so glad that I could breathe again. I was hoping the fear was gone and I could move on.

It's hard to imagine how the word Cancer effects people. Instantly they think they will catch it. Everyone fears it. You thought you had friends, you did while you were on sick leave, there were phone calls and cards and reminders of how much you were missed. When I went back to work I could see people looking at me from a distance, no way were they going to come to welcome me back. I did my job as best I could, ate my lunch in my car and was just glad to be alive. I never acted any different towards the people, I understood their fear.

When you are diagnosed with Cancer your whole world changes, all of a sudden you want to do everything, go every where eat everything that you hadn't eaten before and just live, live, live. There is no stopping you. You have a terrible fear that you will not live another day. I became familiar with alcohol, I liked the way it made me feel, I forgot about the Cancer, chemo, radiation and doctors. I was enjoying life, I changed my hair, my clothes, my makeup my whole attitude, I was doing things that I never had done before, and I was liking it. I knew it wasn't good to be drinking while doing the treatment, but I did not care. I was going to enjoy life, and I did.

Things look different, food smells different, even the air smells different, you see things different, like the sun rise and sunset, you really take time to notice everything even a small ant crawling on the ground, a bird singing in the morning and how good the rain feels on your face, and you no longer run to get out of it. You see life so different. One thing that I totally hated was television, it was constantly talking about Cancer treatment centers, that was the last thing I wanted to hear. I knew the commericals were on television before, I guess I just didn't notice it as much, but now I had this problem and it was very upsetting almost like it was haunting me. I noticed more people with disabilities, people in wheel chairs, the old and the young, everything a constant reminder of my illness. I was sick but I knew if I kept on fighting I just might survive again.

Check ups were mandatory, if you wanted to keep ahead of the disease, it was always waiting to strike again, and it did. When I went back for a check up, I was hoping to hear the word remission, the only thing I heard was you now have a tumor in your right kidney, and it will require six more months of chemo, and they would be installing a wire shunt into my kidney to keep it open. If the Cancer returned it would probably hit my spleen, they were insistent about removing it," I said no." It was in my kidney and had totally missed my spleen, it wasn't even on the same side of my body. I was so relieved that I didn't let them take it out. Sometimes I wondered if they even knew what they were doing. I never did hear the word remission, I guess it wasn't even in their vocabulary.

The good news was after five years and no new occurrences you could consider yourself cured. So as the years pass you push the thought of Cancer to the back of your mind, you try to live your life and every day thank God that you made it this far. I was having positive thoughts, my doctor visits were further apart. three months, six months, once a year until you get to the three year mark. This period lasted from 1993 until 1997.

The doctor is always telling you to keep weight on just in case you get sick again, the last time I lost eighty one pounds. As each year passes you tend to breathe a little easier even though every ache and pain reminds you that the Cancer can be back, your heart races your palms sweats and your fear is unleashed again. The body is never the same, you can always remember how your body felt before the chemo and radiation and you keep hoping that some day the old body will return, but it doesn't. You will have so many aches and pains in your joints, and all you will want to do is sit, because it hurts too bad to move or walk. You get joint pain, your muscles ache, especially when it is going to rain. Your nerves has twinges, like sharp electric zaps, you can develop blood clots, be put on blood thinners, take a chemo that causes needles to go through your hands, face and body if exposed to the cold.

No matter what you are told about chemo and radiation, if you experience it you will never ever forget it.

Chapter Seven

The Year 2000

In 2000, my mother passed away without warning, my brother and I were devastated, she was to have a simple heart operation, everything went as planned, she had to go to Washington, D.C. for the surgery. I lived in Baltimore, Bill came to my house and we went to the hospital together. When we arrived she had decided she didn't want to have the surgery, we felt it was her choice so it had been agreed.

We left her room to get some lunch and take a break. When we returned she had changed her mind and was ready to have the surgery. To this day we still don't know why she decided to have the surgery. She was really ready to do it.

During surgery something went wrong and she never survived. The doctors informed us her heart and lungs froze up, they don't know what happened to cause this. We were so shocked, that the operation failed and she had died. She had such a positive attitude about the surgery. If she would have went with her first instinct she may have lived. My mom would call me every Sunday and we would catch up, we live about 150 miles apart. I was never allowed to talk about my illness, she never believed I was sick.

I never thought my mother accepted my illness, she couldn't believe I had Cancer because no one before me in the family had it. She never came to visit me in all the years that I dealt with it. She always told me the doctors were quacks, they didn't know what they were talking about. When my father was killed in the automobile accident no one ever knew his health issues, back then records were not kept like they are now. My father could have been the carrier of the Cancer gene. I guess we will never know.

I had also moved back to my hometown where my brother was living, my kids were grown and had kids, he had grown kids and grand kids too, so I thought it would be nice to get out of the city, move back to the country, I could transfer my job so that was good. Bill and I weren't really close because we had lived so far apart for all those years but I knew once I moved back to Western Maryland we could pick up where we left off when we were kids. Bill helped me move back home.

I went back to work working for the same company only in a different location. I liked my job so that made things easier with the move. I found a really nice apartment in a nice neighborhood and started to adjust to my new lifestyle. Life was quiet here and I really didn't miss the noise and confusion of the big city, it was a little like heaven here. While shopping one day I ran into my old friend Trecia, it was great to see her, She hadn't changed much in thirty years, we still recognized each other. She hadn't married and was still as crazy as ever. Our friendship had never changed we were still best friends. We had so much catching up to do. She had been involved in quite a few relationships and apparently none of them worked out, I guess that was why she was still single. She wasn't the marrying type anyway. She seemed happy and that was all that mattered.

One day over coffee and coke a cola, she drank coffee, I never liked it, we got talking about living expenses and how hard it was to make it on your own.

The suggestion came up about sharing living expenses, my apartment was small, one bedroom, but really nice and so was hers, together we were paying out double, why not get a bigger place and share the expenses. It was the best thing we ever did and we could save money too. We got along well and things I thought were starting to look up.

Chapter Eight

The Year 2004

In the Spring of 2004 I had developed a severe cold, which I couldn't shake. When I went to the doctors in May I was given cough syrup and antibiotics. I took the medicine until it was gone, but the symptoms were still there, I still couldn't breathe right, I felt I wasn't getting any better, so the doctor decided to change the medication. I had quit smoking earlier that month. I had smoked for at least 35 years when finally with the help of Trecia, I threw them away. I am now smoke free it has been six wonderful years. Even with me giving up smoking I wasn't feeling any better.

One day while watching television, I was sitting on my couch when a rather large lump appeared under my right jaw line next to my ear, it was about the size of a fifty cent piece. I asked Trecia what do you think about this? She reminded me that I had a doctors appointment the next day and she suggested I discuss it with him.

The doctor was checking it out but he wasn't quite sure what it was. I asked if it could be the lymphoma again since it was so close to my lymph nodes I always had a sixth sense about the Cancer, I always knew when it was back. Not wanting to make any kind of a statement, he set me up an appointment with an ear, nose and throat specialist.

Upon my visit to the ear, nose and throat doctor it was determined I had Cancer on my right tonsil. He decided to remove the bad tonsil and left the other one in there, I was referred to Morgantown University

Hospital home of the West Virginia School of Medicine. They were going to do an evaluation on me. West Virginal Medical School was quite sure that I had the Cancer again. So it began all over, the testing, blood work, cat scans, mri's, biopsies and now a new machine called a pet scan, it was like an mri only it scanned your body all the way through from front to back, clear through, missing nothing not even a mole.

After all the testing was finished, I got the good news again, "yes you have it and this kind is squamous cell and it is located in the right side of your neck". I knew that lump wasn't good. Great just what I wanted to hear, immediately my past life with the chemo and radiation flashed in my brain, did I really want to put up with that misery again. They did some more testing and they found a small spot on the roof of my mouth, it too was Cancerous. This one was called single cell. Both Cancers were in stage four, this is when it is metastasized, this means it has invaded other parts of the body. Stage four is also the last stage before death.

The doctors tried to explain all that was involved, it didn't sound easy to me, there was so much surgery, they were going to do things to me that had never been done before. Did I want to be a guinea pig for this school? I knew it was going to be difficult, but I had no other choice, if I didn't have the surgery I was told I had six weeks to live. I wish now that I never had it done, just how long could I have lived, well I guess I will never know. I didn't feel bad, I only had a cold.

The surgery would take at least fifteen hours (can you imagine?) with no guarantees and my case would have to be presented before a board of surgeons to see if it would be approved, because it was so extreme. This was October 2004.

I went home talked to my kids, my brother and my friends, to explain the situation, they told me I was strong and I would make it, I had made it three other times, this wouldn't be any different. Little did I realize the extent of it all. What ever happened to the third time is the charm?

On the morning of November 1st 2004, I was as ready as I ever would be. I was scared to death, but I knew God and my friends would take care of me.

The surgeons consisted of the ear, nose and throat doctor, orthopedic doctors and multiple students specializing in the field of Cancer. I felt pretty safe. After fifteen hours of being on the operating table Dr. Vanders told my family and friends, it would be okay to go home and return in the morning because was I resting quietly.

I was put into an induced coma for three days, and I had a tracheotomy, this was something I never had before, and I had a tube in my stomach.

The surgery would consist of taking out my pallet, (because of the Cancer in the roof of my mouth) lymph nodes from my neck, a fibula bone from out of my left leg to make a bridge in my mouth so I could wear my teeth, and skin grafts to make a covering for the hole that would be left in my mouth after they removed my pallet. the surgery ended up being more evasive than they realized.

I now had no pallet, they had removed twenty lymph nodes from my neck and removed my shoulder muscle which I had not been informed of, my fibula bone from my leg, they took skin grafts from my upper leg. (two grafts) Something happened to my right ear, after I came home I noticed my hearing was failing in my right ear. I was positioned in my room so that I couldn't see myself in the mirror. I had my own personal nurse so I knew I must have looked pretty bad. With my pallet gone, I couldn't swallow right or breathe right, the hole was just a passage and it let in too much air. The doctor installed a mouth piece that a football player would wear to protect his teeth while playing football to my upper gums and he had to put it in with screws so that it wouldn't come out, it hurt so bad.

Chapter Nine

Thirteen Days

Three days after waking from the self induced coma, I was groggy and so out of it I wasn't functioning like I should be, It was hard for me to make sense out of anything. I was becoming aware that I had a feeding tube in my nose, a drain tube in the right side of my neck, a breathing tube in my mouth a trach in my throat, a rubber football mouth piece, drains in my left leg and of course IV's in my arm. It made me wonder what they really did to me. I kept wondering if I was alive. For a brief moment I remembered someone talking to me, they were assuring me that I would be fine, I didn't recognize the voices until my kids, Bill my brother and Trecia told me it was them. I felt some relief at least I knew I was alive. I don't remember any pain, I'm sure they had given me the maximum dosage of what ever it took to keep me pain free, I sure don't remember asking for anything for pain.

Trying to give me a bath was almost impossible, the nurses had to put their arms under the back of my head while the other washed my hair, I remember when they washed it and they washed it several times, the first time they rinsed it the water ran red with blood. It too was making me wonder why I had so much blood in my hair, when I asked why, the answer was it was from the operation. (did I have any blood left) The bath was just as bad, they had to move all the tubes and lines so that they could wash me, it wasn't a pleasant experience.

I was glad when the bath was over. I was completely confused by everything that was going on. I didn't understand why I couldn't look in the mirror. I had a million questions racing through my head, and no answers.

The very thought of all this was making me ill, I didn't know what to think of it. I had went to sleep and was awaken by some kind of an alarm. I had pulled all the tubes out of me, the food tube, the drain tubes, breathing tubes and even the IV's, the blood was squirting every where, each time my heart would pump, the blood would fly. I was a total mess, of course they put all of the tubes back in without taking me to surgery, they just started forcing them back in, I sure hoped I didn't pull them out again, that wasn't very pleasant.

The football piece that had been screwed into my top gum kept coming out because they didn't have anything to attach it to. The right side was completely gone, there was no place to attach it, it would stay hooked to the left side until I bit down and then it came loose. There was nothing in my mouth except a large hole. How can you attach anything to a hole? I was able to put a false plate of teeth in and it held as long as I kept my mouth shut. Not only did I have trouble with the top plate, I couldn't open my mouth far enough to get the bottom teeth in, for some reason my jaw was now locked and I could only open it about an inch to an inch and a half. With them taking twenty lymph nodes out of my neck and removing my shoulder muscle the jaw tightened up and I could no longer get my mouth open and no longer wear my teeth.

I no longer had a pallet on my right side and they also had to reposition my nose, if they had left it the way it was, my nose would have caved in and my nose would have been off center either to the right or left, they weren't sure which way it would go. Thank God they did get that right.

I was having trouble eating, they tried giving me soft foods, like mashed potatoes, puddings, and applesauce. I had a hard time drinking too. The nurses were with me 24 hours a day, I was still in the critical care unit, and I still hadn't looked in a mirror. Since the incident where I pulled out the plugs and lines they kept a male nurse with me at all times. I figured they thought I would do it again and I just may have.

Several days after the surgery the nurses came into my room to change my leg bandage, I hadn't seen this operation yet where they had removed my fibula bone. This is the most expandable bone in the body and they were going to use it for a new bridge in my mouth. I was so shocked when they removed the bandage that I almost passed out. I know the blood had to drain out of my face, and probably out of my body. The size of the cut was amazing, it had to have been at least ten to eleven inches in length and at least five to six inches in diameter, it was from the bottom of my knee reaching to my ankle, I was so shocked that I couldn't even speak. If I hadn't known better I would have sworn that I had been bitten by a shark, that is exactly what it looked like. It didn't look like a surgery it actually looked like my leg had been bitten. Why such a large area, I know the bridge in my mouth could only have been six inches doubled, then I notice the upper part of my left leg, in two different places they were bandaged also, this was where they took the skin graphs to use to cover the hole in my mouth. The bandages on the skin graphs would remain on my leg until I was released from the hospital.

The surgeon came in to visit me and to see how I was doing. He made an apology concerning the operation, It had taken too much time and they were losing me on the table after fifteen hours, they didn't have time to complete the operation, apparently they had done the skin grafts and the removal of the fibula bone first, when they got into removing the Cancer in my mouth, Cancer in my neck, removing the twenty lymph nodes and my shoulder muscle there must not have been time to install the bridge in my mouth and cover the hole with the skin graphs. The doctor informed me that they had such a difficult time with the muscle in my leg, I have always worked on my feet and my legs were very muscular, he went on to tell me that once they cut the skin and removed the fibula bone which the muscle adheres to, the muscle wouldn't stay intact. They had to use the skin graft from the upper part of my leg to cover the opening and to keep the muscle in. I had clamps and stitches all the way around where they had removed the bone. I had two patches of skin covering it. It had a drain tube also.

Within the next couple of days they had me walking, it was really hard to balance myself even with the walker, you are so afraid that your leg is going to break because you know the bone that helps you walk and keeps your leg straight is gone.

I was just glad that my recovery in the hospital was going well, and I was ready to go home. My walking had improved and as far as eating most of it was going in to the trash. I was informed that I couldn't go home until I was able to eat. I wasn't going to stay any longer than I had to. It was almost impossible to get anything down so I improvised the situation and fed the garbage can. I fed it enough that I was going home. I was the happiest person on the planet.

Right before I was to be released, one of the students came in to change the bandage on my upper leg where I had the skin graphs, when he started removing it I was in tears not only did it hurt but when he pulled it off the bandage stuck, he just continued to pull it very fast I thought this is worse than any pain I had endured since I have been here. My skin felt like it was being ripped off, like it was on fire. Finally it was over and I was going home.

I was so glad to still be alive, but what I had endured was only the beginning of the real recovery process.

Chapter Ten

Recovering

As we drove out of the hospital I was never so glad to be saying goodbye to that house of horrors. As I looked back at it all I could see was the horrible experience that I had just went through, it wasn't over yet, this was now the beginning, and besides in two weeks I had to return for my first check up.

The drive home was long and enduring, I realize it was only 70 miles but I was so weak and distraught that all I wanted to do was get home. I didn't want to look in the car mirror, so I would wait until I got home and got settled, I would soon find out why they kept hiding the mirror from me. Bill was waiting for us when we arrived, he was there to help me get into the house, I had four steps to climb and then a landing, he wanted to try and carry me and I said no way, just balance the walker on each step and I could pull myself up. It worked great, I had no trouble at all. Getting into the house was easier than I thought. Going back down the steps would probably he harder, oh well I wasn't going to think about that for two weeks.

I had noticed on the ride home the noise didn't seem right, you know how the wind makes noise when you're riding, I noticed the sound in my right ear was different, this again was the side I had all the surgery on, it was like I couldn't hear the wind. I even wound down the window a little and again no sound. I couldn't image what had happened to my hearing. I thought it would clear up.

After Bill left the first thing I wanted to see was my face, I was horrified, I had a scar from under my right ear all the way under my chin and ended in the middle of my throat, it had to be at least eight inches in length. The right side of my neck was gone and the right side of my face was swollen also. I took the small compact mirror and looked in my mouth and all I saw looking back at me was a large hole that covered the whole right upper portion of my mouth. It was sickening, I could feel my stomach churning. No wonder they wouldn't let me have a mirror. They probably knew I would have became angry in the hospital. It was just so hard to look at my face and neck now and remember what I looked like before I went in for the surgery. I had no idea what they were going to do to me, and that I would look like I do now. Being alive was the only thing that kept me going, really I had no other choice but to make the best of it.

I had a terrible time eating and drinking. I couldn't swallow the food it would go up into the hole and then I would choke, I couldn't drink, and I had a really hard time chewing, I had no way to keep my teeth in I was just a mess. I soon found out the reason I chocked so much was because they had removed my saliva glands, these are the glands that produce saliva which is the liquid in your mouth that helps you swallow. I no longer had these glands so my food what I could get in my mouth was always dry. I found out if I would take a drink and wet my mouth first it would be easier to swallow the food. I had to eat everything soft. I knew I was losing weight but I couldn't help it, who in their right mind would want to live this way, I was practically a vegetable. We had to change the bandages on my leg once a day and every time we would remove the dressing I would get sick again. We had to buy special bandages that already had some kind of lubricant on them for the incision where they had removed the fibula bone, the upper skin graphs just took regular bandages.

My ear was still closed off and I couldn't hear anything. I would tell them when I went back to the hospital.

The two weeks had arrived already and it was time to go back for my check up. Dr. Vanders was glad to see me and reminded me I was looking really well. He was such a kind doctor. I felt a little better when he said I looked good. I thought "boy the other patients must really look bad." He did an examination and while he was informing me of different things his students were standing by observing his every move. He then asked me if there was anything wrong and I explained about my ear. He informed me he thought there might be ear damage because of the surgery being so close to my ear, sometimes it happens and sometimes it don't. Of course it had to happen to me. While I was sitting in the chair he told me he would install a tube in the ear canal and this would hold it open and I would be able to hear again. The instant he installed the little tube in my ear, I could hear. He also informed me that I may have to have it done more than once. Your body will reject anything that is foreign. Dr. Vanders also told me how sorry he was about the surgery, they just couldn't go on because they didn't want to lose me, and it should have been done in two parts. They were going to do it that way at first but felt it would take too much of a toll on me.

He knew I couldn't go back to work and so he insisted on putting me on medical disability, every thing was taken care of then and there, all I had to do was take the papers to the disability board and I would be approved.

When I returned home I went to the disability office and had every thing taken care of. The next trip would be to the Cancer Center for my evaluation. I couldn't wait, After going through it twice before I was thrilled to be there. I was treated great, the staff was very kind. They explained what I had in store for me and how much treatment I would have to have. The results were to be thirty five treatments of radiation, no chemo, thank God again. I would have the treatment in the upper right side of my face. They designed a mask for me to wear while doing the treatment. You have to cover the exposed area or it will be damaged. My treatment was to start in two weeks.

Come Monday morning at 9:00 a.m. I would arrive, I was still using the walker and I was getting along with it pretty good. I still didn't have any strength in my leg. I could put it down but only for a few seconds. When the blood ran down into my leg, it would thump and thump.

Although Dr. Vanders told me they got all the Cancer, I would still have to do treatment just in case it could come back so quick after the surgery. the radiation was to prevent it.

The two weeks passed quickly and I wasn't really looking forward to the treatment, but I knew it had to be done, so off I went to the Cancer Center to get started. Thirty five treatments would take thirty five trips once a day. The treatments took about 20 minutes each time I went, and I knew with each treatment I would grow weaker. I had all hopes that things might go good this time. Please Lord give me the strength to endure this treatment. This was my prayer each and every time I would get ready to go out the door.

Chapter Eleven

Treatment

I knew what was in store for me when I opened the door to the Cancer Center, It hadn't changed any. I would be interviewed by the Cancer Specialist, asked a million questions, give a million answers, then came the explanation of what they were going to do and how they would do it.

I was only receiving radiation no chemo this time, and they would be positioning it to hit my cheek. It was like a laser that you see on tv. The treatment took about twenty minutes to complete. With chemo it took hours sometimes three to four.

The first one wasn't so bad, I felt okay except for the burning in my cheek, I noticed it was red and so was the inside of my mouth. The radiation had penetrated through the whole right side of my face. I always wondered how they determined the amount of radiation to give to someone, did everyone get the same amount? This was never discussed. This was only the first treatment and I started feeling sick on my stomach. I always ate Nabisco saltine crackers when I was sick from the other chemo and radiation treatments. I didn't know if the radiation caused it or it was the thought of going through the treatments again. I only had thirty four more to go. When I left the center I noticed how drained I felt, I was hoping when I got home I could rest and try to eat something. Soup was about the only thing I could consume, except for liquid nutritional supplements and they tasted horrible, the staff was always saying try this, try that, they would even give them to you, Ensure and Boost, no I just couldn't get them down and everything else was too hard to eat.

I finally finished the first week and I was so glad that I had two days off. I noticed my mouth was starting to get sore. The doctor had given me a special kind of mouth wash, I was to use it before I ate, it was was to numb my mouth so I could eat. That was great except I couldn't taste the food. It did numb my mouth so eating was a little less painful. I just really took it easy on my two days off, and I so looked forward to holidays because I knew the center would be closed then too. For every holiday the Cancer Center would erect a tree for that occasion, if it was Halloween, they would have a tree full of pumpkins and ghost. I often wondered if they did the tree thing in case you didn't make it to the next holiday. Death was always on your mind. When you would go for treatment and look at the other souls you felt even worse. The trips to West Virginia University to see Dr. Vanders was the most devastating, You got to see all the surgical patients all in one room waiting to see the doctors, it just looked like a chop shop for humans. You knew in your heart these people went under the knife to save their lives and now they looked like people in horror movies. I saw one man there that had a scar similar to mine, his neck was cut like mine but his face had a scar from the center of his nose to the left ear. He wasn't an old person either, I'd say he may have been in his forties. Cancer doesn't discriminate, no matter what sex you are or age, if you are on its list, it is coming for you.

It was time to go back to West Virginia again for my check up. Things were going good so far except I was still having trouble keeping my teeth in. Dr. Vanders recommended that I see their dentist who was also a teaching physician at WV. They were able to get me in that day so I wouldn't have to make another trip down. The doctor was very kind, he explained what he would do to my teeth so that they would stay intact. The dentist took an impression of my gums and of course the giant hole in the roof of my mouth. He assured me he could do something to help me. On the right side of my upper plate he built up a mound exactly the size of the hole. When I inserted the teeth in my mouth it filled the hole completely and closed off all air from passing through. I felt better already. I could even smile without my teeth falling out, like I had anything to smile about. I could no longer wear my bottom teeth because my jaw was locked. At least when I got home would I be able to eat? It felt weird at first but it actually worked. I kept seeing a commericial on television about K.F.C. pot pies.

For some reason I wanted one so badly, I became addicted to Kentucky Fried Chicken's pot pies, they were something new and I wanted to try them. I was hooked the first time I tried them, they were soft and easy to swallow, and of course I was getting my meat and vegetables, the sauce on them helped me to swallow them with ease. I know I ate them every day for at least two months. They filled the void in my food chain and I could actually eat them with no trouble at all. The dentist at WV. had made my life a lot better. I was so thankful to him.

By now I was about half way through my treatment and I started to notice a build up of white blisters forming on the inside of my mouth. I wasn't sure what they were so when I returned to do treatment on Monday I asked to speak with the doctor and she informed me they were blisters from the radiation, "great just what I wanted to hear." She gave me medication to help clear them up. It was almost impossible to get rid of them because every time I ate, the medicine was dissolved. I was only eating one meal a day and now I had blisters to deal with. Each time I would eat the blisters would become more severe, the pain was terrible, Did you ever have a blister on your heel from new shoes? Just imagine a whole mouth full of them. I could barely get the food moved around in my mouth to chew it. I know sometimes I was swallowing whole pieces of food because I couldn't chew it, my next fear: "What if I choke'?

After each meal whether it would be liquid or solid I would have to clean my mouth, take the teeth out, clean the hole and all around my mouth, I used at least ten cotton swabs each time I cleaned it, even with the hole blocked food was able to get in it at times, especially soft foods, like mashed potatoes. They were a real problem, sometimes they would cause me to choke.

I started eating less and less and then I started losing weight. It was just so hard to eat with the blisters and I couldn't get them cleared up because the radiation keep coming. The radiation was actually burning me on the inside and outside. I had developed busted blood vessels on my cheek. The inside of my right jaw to this day still stays red and inflamed looking.

I still had ten treatments to do twenty-five gone, I was over half way there, I knew I would make it but the blisters were still unbearable. I talked to the doctor and she suggested I take some time off and try to get the blisters healed before I continued the radiation. This was good. I did every thing to get the blisters healed, I didn't eat spicy things or hot things crunchy things or anything that I knew would irritate the blisters. I took it slow and for the two weeks that I didn't have treatment I felt good again.

I kept thinking only ten more could I make it? Sooner than I thought it was time to return to do it all again. The blisters had almost healed and I was feeling better, maybe I could get done with the treatments before they acted up again. I was almost finished with the walker, I had been walking on my own at home and I was doing pretty good. The surgery on my leg had healed almost over, it still had left a horrible scar, one that no one would be proud of. I would wear pants, no more shorts for me, and probably now I would be wearing long dresses. I didn't want people staring at me and asking "what happened to your leg"? Trecia and Bill suggested that I tell people it was a shark bite, amazing enough that's exactly what it looked like.

The rest of the treatment went pretty well, and I knew by the time I finished it I would have the blisters back. I was still losing weight and it was coming off pretty fast, I tried to eat but it was almost impossible again. Five more to go. I was actually dragging (with help) myself into the center just so I could get the last treatments done. I will never know how I made it this far. Finally the last day of treatment came and I was ready to get it over with. Surprise! When we got to the center for treatment we were informed that the radiation machine was broke down and it may be two hours before it was up and running. Wonderful, just what I wanted to hear. I looked at the nurse and I said "you better get it fixed, because if I have to leave here today without the treatment I will not be back." We waited for about twenty minutes and I was informed that the machine was working again, God must have been looking out for me. I did my treatment and when I was leaving they gave me a puppet that looked like a flower, a certificate of graduation for completing the treatment and many many hugs. I was so weak I could barely walk out of that place, by this time I had lost sixty pounds. I put my butt in high gear and although I was as slow as a snail I made the transition to the outside world. It was over and I knew in my heart I would never go through it again.

Chapter Twelve

Physical Therapy

Radiation treatment was finally over, now I was hoping I could rest for a while. Wrong, now I had to start going to physical therapy so that I could learn to walk right without falling and stumbling like I was drunk, and how to use my arm and shoulder where they had removed the twenty lymph nodes and my shoulder muscle, I could clearly see there was no rest. The doctor informed me the quicker I got back on my feet the better I would feel, yeah it was easy for him to say, I could barely move let alone walk after the radiation. I needed to take a break and that is just what I did.

One month after taking the break, getting the blisters cleared up in my mouth and I was beginning to feel like eating again, I decided to take the doctors up on the therapy. I was still eating the pot pies, it was like I was addicted to them, they were so good and I was so thankful that the restaurant was so close.

While opening my mail, I came upon a statement from the insurance company. They always send you a copy of what they paid and what your balance was. Thank God I didn't owe anything I had already reached my deductible so my insurance company had to pay the balance. I almost fainted when I saw the bill for the surgery at West Virginia University, are you ready?

$369,000.00. I was so glad I didn't have to pay it, how could I have paid it? There was no way. I bet this money put a few students through medical school. I hope they were the ones that had watched my surgery. The physical therapy wasn't too awful. I was still weak but I tried doing what they asked. They would stimulate my arm with some kind of electric shock to awaken the nerves so that it would work better, it did actually work very well, until I went home and the stimulation stopped. I walked pretty good before starting the therapy. They would show me how to balance myself by walking between a balance beam, both hands on the bars, but when I let go, I was like a ship that had too much cargo on one side I would tilt. This whole ordeal was pretty frustrating, but I knew if I wanted to get better and stronger I would have to follow along.

The therapy lasted about six weeks and when I left I was walking better, my shoulder was stronger, my arms were stronger, they sent me home with a device that you could hang on your door, you could pull it up and down, this was to make my shoulder stronger. I didn't understand how it would work considering I didn't have any muscle in my shoulder to build up. They said if I used it, it would help. I still have movement in my shoulder, but if I want to reach up for something I had to push my arm up with my left arm and hold it in position until I could reach the object, it just won't lift up on its own.

I was glad the therapy was over, now maybe I could relax. I was still traveling to West Virginia to see Dr. Vanders for my monthly visit. I noticed once again my hearing wasn't as good as before. By driving at higher elevations it seemed different. He had explained that the tube may work itself out without me knowing it. While I was there I had him check it again, Yep it was missing, he said he could reinstall one, but this time he was going to let one of his students do it. Big mistake, the girl was so shaky and nervous and I was going through so much pain because she couldn't get it positioned in the right place. She must have poked me every where except where she was suppose to, I was ready to jump out of the chair and deck her. Dr. Vanders came in to check on me and he noticed that I was in so much pain that I was crying, he excused her and he took over and finished installing the tube. Between the male student ripping the bandages off of my leg before I went home from the surgery and this girl poking me like a pin cushion I was ready to give up on this hospital.

He apologized for thinking she was ready to undertake this most important task. My visits to WV. became father and father apart, I had been going every two weeks, then once a month and now it was going to be every six months. I was sick of traveling that long road back and forth and now I wouldn't have to do it so often.

I was determined to return to work, there was no way I could live on the disability I was getting. My expenses were more than the income. Mentally and physically I wanted to try to work again. I set up an appointment with Dr. Vanders and explained the situation to him. He felt that because of my leg not having a bone in it, it would be hard for me to be on my feet for a long period of time. Of course my job was being on my feet. He felt my leg may give out, but if I wanted it that bad it would be my decision. He suggested I give it a try and he would stand by me. Before I had the surgery he told me I may never work again. I went to disability and informed them of what I wanted to do. Of course they were shocked, people just didn't give up their disability, After I explained the situation they agreed if I wanted to try it, go for it. If it didn't work out I could always reapply. They would continue to give me the disability check for a year to see if I could do the job, if I couldn't do the job then I would already be in the system and I wouldn't have to reapply.

I got all the necessary paper work done, I knew I could only be off on sick leave for a year and a day, if I was off longer I would lose my position and I would have to start over. I had worked too hard to get to where I was in the company; there was no turning back now.

While I was on sick leave I would go to my job to visit my friends. First I went in a wheel chair, then with a walker and then I walked in on my own. My friends were always glad to see me. I was like a celebrity. They were so amazed how I had gone through what I had and still survived, not one of them thought I would make it, nor did I. I had left work on October 21, 2004, had the surgery on November 1, 2004, came home on November 13th, 2004, started radiation therapy in December of 2004, finished it in February of 2004, started physical therapy in March of 2004, finished it in May of 2004. Now I was ready to start a new life. I had everything going for me now, I was going to enjoy the summer rebuild my life and return to work on October 22, 2004.

Chapter Thirteen

Back to Work

During the Summer of 2005, I got a lot accomplished. I felt better, I could walk better and I could go places without taking my little friend along. He was standing home alone and not walking with me. It took a long time for me to start to feel better about things. I was very self conscious about my neck and face. When someone would talk to me I would turn my head so that they wouldn't look at me. Every where I went I felt like I was being stared out. My friends kept telling me it didn't look that bad, but they weren't the one that had to go through it. In my mind I thought I looked totally different. When you are use to looking one way and then you look another you can notice it. My looks hadn't changed that much it was the scars that I was left with. How was I going to go back to work in a public place where I had to deal with people all the time. I decided to grow my hair longer, at least it would cover part of my neck. It was hard for me to wear makeup, for some reason the chemicals in the makeup would cause the nerves in my face to react, and applying the makeup was almost impossible because I couldn't rub my skin, it would set the nerves off, I couldn't wear any kind of jewelry especially earrings, I just could not get them to quit hurting when I put them in my right ear, I even tried ones with no posts (clip ons) I could wear them in my left, but forget the right. I could only wear a necklace for a short and then it would rub my neck and cause the nerves to become irritated. I had always worn a chain that had a mermaid on it, a small birthstone ring, and a little trinket that said #1 Mom. My son Willie had given them to me a long time ago. The mermaid I found on the floor of a bar while I was doing the wild thing with the Cancer. My biggest fear was how people would look at me, would they accept me, or look the other way, or just ignore it? I needed to get my mind made up, was I going to be able to handle this? I have always been a private person and now I was going to be in the limelight.

On October 22, 2005 I walked through the doors of my old job. My first concern was will I be able to work for eight hours. I had to try. I felt the same about my friends when I returned and I thought they felt the same about me. I noticed people acted shy around me, like they didn't know how to approach me or what to talk about. These were the same people that were hugging me when I would come for a visit. What happened? I really believe they never thought I would come back to work. I think a lot of them thought I was going to die by the way I looked when I came to the store for a visit. Even my best friends (so I thought) acted the same way. They must have thought they could catch the Cancer. I just didn't understand the whole situation. Even the manager of the store made a statement to me, "why didn't you just stay on disability? I was shocked that he made that comment. Was he really being concerned or was he ashamed that I came back? I knew I had to work so I did the best that I could do. I explained to him disability was not an option, I couldn't make it on that little bit of money. (I do not understand how people survive on disability.)

I was placed in groceries, doing everything, it was a consumable department and it was constantly replenished, it kept me hopping, but if you knew me you would know I was doing good and keeping up. Each day was a new challenge, when I would go home at night I wouldn't move off the couch until it was time for bed. Once I had returned to work I noticed a difference in my hearing again. Instead of going back to WV. I got a referral here with an ear, nose and throat doctor. I was so glad. Dr. Nova said he would have to replace the tube again, this was the third time I have had this procedure. He told me the tube only last about a year. I was just happy to hear again, and I thought well another year another tube.

I stayed in groceries for about fourteen months, just when I got use to it, I was moved to tire, and lube express, this was more like working in a garage, we sold oil, tires, all kinds of grease, air freshner devices, anything to do with cars, we had the department that changed tires and oil too. My friend (whom I had been his department manager when I first started there in automotive) James was now my supervisor, he never ever treated me any different. He and I had been friends for a long time, he was my night shelf stalker in automotive and he did a great job. When the tire and lube department managers position came open, I suggested to him to apply for it since he was already familiar with the department, and since it was an off spring of automotive, the only difference they would be doing tire and oil changes, I knew he could handle that. That's how he became my boss in tire and lube. We worked great together, just like in the other department.

I worked in the tire and lube for twelve months until James got the axe. I tried to warn him that something wasn't right, they were constantly riding him about things. I felt like they were setting him up. They had it out for him anyway and I guess they moved me there to help him get organized, he was at the point where he didn't care anymore, I tried to help him, but he wasn't giving an inch. Eventually they fired him. I missed him a lot, he was a good worker, I just don't think he was management material. He had always worked for me. On a scale of one to ten, he was an eleven. "Wonder where I go next."
This was now the second month of 2008.

Kim was a small auburn haired girl with red highlights, she was currently managing cosmetics, she was a special friend to me and had always treated me great. She too was sick a lot, she had went through much testing too, to try and find out what her problems were. It had something to do with her lungs, she always had problems even as a child with breathing, of course she had been a smoker but when all the testing started she had quit. Finally she was diagnosed with cystic fibrosis, it was in curable and her only option was a lung transplant. Kim would have to give up her job and she would have to move to Florida where they would preform the transplant if one became available. I was asked to take over the cosmetic department. It was one of the worst departments in the store, it had so many, many small items, like lipstick, perfume, eye makeup, eye shadow, powder, face creams, anything to do with being beautiful. This is just what I wanted a department where I should be looking good and I looked like hell. Was this a slur to my face? After the remark the manager made to me, It made me wonder. At first I really felt out of place, I knew women would be coming into this department and asking me questions about makeup and how they looked and I'm sure they would notice how I looked. I was a good one to advise them, me looking like I had arrived from a horror flick. I put my whole life into it and kept thinking how bad off Kim was. If she didn't get a donor, she would probably die. I would do my best to keep her department running smooth. I would make her proud. She always told me I was a good worker.

Kim had been in Florida for over a year waiting for a transplant, and finally it happened, there was a donor. Everyone was so happy for her, she had been through so much, she had to give up her life to live. We were all praying for her. The news we received wasn't good, she didn't survive the operation. We didn't know what happened, she just didn't make it. My heart sank, I knew her well and only wished the best for her. This was just another disappointment in my life. It has been a year since she passed away and she is and always will be in our prayers.

The cosmetic department was so huge and so complicated, at the end of the day I was really ready to go home and just pull my hair out. It was the hardest department that I had ever worked in.

One thing good the customers never made a comment about my looks, if they asked about my condition, I knew it was out of concern, they seem so thoughtful. They would share their stories of a friend or family member that had been ill. My fears of people judging me on my appearance cleared up. People were not making me feel uncomfortable like I thought they would, they were very sympathetic.

Actually I was enjoying working the department, I was able to see all the new kinds of makeup and would try different things to see how my face would respond. If I used a very light foundation it worked pretty well, with the foundation and mascara I was set to go. I never wore any kind of lip stick or lip balms so I didn't have to worry about that.

I thought I was doing a very good job but apparently management didn't. No matter which way I would turn they were after me for something. (In the back of my mind I felt like James, I knew what they did to him.) I had been a department manager for this store for fifteen years and now my head was on the chopping block. I was confused, I didn't know quite what they were looking for, I just felt they were out to get me. I was a dedicated employee, I was always on time, I only missed work if I was sick, I never took unnecessary breaks or lunches. I gave this company 110 %. Was It because I was ill and the insurance company was tired of paying for me?. As hard as I tried to step down from the department the more road blocks I encountered. No matter what I did, there was no new jobs available, or so I was told. What had I done to deserve this kind of treatment, something was wrong. Finally after eighteen months I said" no more." I went to the manager and asked one more time to step down. I knew he had to give me another job. I knew I would be a regular employee with no title except associate, and I would lose money, but it was either that or lose my mind. I couldn't afford to lose my job, so it was do or die time. Maybe my health would improve.

My ear tube had come out again and I would have to go to Dr. Nova to have it replaced. It would be same day surgery. When he replaced the tube he informed me this one should last forever. I certainly hope so because I am so tired of this too. No wonder people get sick with all the stress we have to endure. The doctors told me this could have been one of the reason that I had developed Cancer so many times.

The stress at work was getting to me and I had to save my health. I sure didn't want Cancer

My new job would be shoes. It was fine, I had to go on nights and no longer had weekends off and I knew I wouldn't be able to sleep during the day, but I wasn't a quitter and they were not going to get the best of me. I mostly worked alone and I liked that. I didn't have to do a lot of paper work, I didn't have to do anything but walk out the door after eight hours. I knew I would make it or die trying. I still had seven years and eight months before I could even think about retiring, that was a long way off, would I get sick again, would my legs hold out, would my arm hold out and my shoulder, every night is a new challenge to walk in to work and just imagine what kind of night I will have. Here we are nine months later April 2010, my new job is shoes I am suppose to be in shoes, but I am working every where in the store doing different jobs. I find it adventures not knowing what I will be doing from night to night. When seven o'clock comes I want to be the first one out the door, but most of the time everyone is in there cars and gone until I get through the store. When I get home my left leg is so swollen that my sock has left an impression around my ankle. My whole body hurts, from head to toe. Even on my two days off the swelling doesn't go down in my leg, it remains swollen all the time. Every day I pray, just let me make it one more day.

It has been Five Years and Three Months since I was lying on the operating table at WVU. It is so unbelievable what has transpired over the last five years. I am so glad to be alive and still able to work, even if Dr. Vanders advised against it. I guess no one knows their own body but themselves. I know I couldn't have stayed at home, It wasn't for me.

You know what I miss most? Singing! I used to sing all the time, I thought I had a pretty good voice, my friends always told me I should make records. Well it's too late now. When I would come home from work I would play the stereo and pretend I was singing at a concert and all the fans were cheering for me. I would sing in my car every where I went. Now with this hole in my mouth and the surgery on my neck and face my voice has changed, I don't even sound the same. When I try to sing I don't have enough air to reach the higher notes. Remember Leann Rymes's song Blue, believe it or not I recorded it on a cassette tape and played it for a friend, they couldn't believe it was me instead of Leann Rymes. I put it in the stereo and played it without their knowledge. They were amazed. I know when I go to heaven I will sing in God's choir and my voice will be restored.

Update April 20, 2010.

Isn't it ironic that sixteen days after finishing this book on Cancer, Easter Sunday, A new lump has appeared on the right side of my neck, it is in the same place that I had the other Cancer. It is about six inches in length. I have been to see a surgeon and he advises me he won't touch it because he says if the lump is removed, I may have to have reconstructed surgery and he cannot perform it. I am still waiting for an appointment at West Virginia University Medical Hospital.

I know God must have something special in store for me because he has kept me around so long. The old saying "God doesn't give you any more than you can handle," makes me feel pretty special, because I think I have handled it all-and then some.

Wanda (Rankin) Lawhorn,
As told to Dr. Tmar.

www.ingramcontent.com/pod-product-compliance
Lightning Source LLC
Chambersburg PA
CBHW050339290526
45785CB00006B/2561